Essential Oils

Quick Start Essential Oils For Beginners And Aromatherapy For Organic Natural Beauty And Health!

Sarah Brooks

Copyright © 2015 Sarah Brooks

STOP!!! Before you read any further....Would you like to know the secrets of Anti-Aging?

If your answer is yes, then you are not alone. Thousands of people are looking for the secret to reducing wrinkles, looking younger, and maintaining a youthful appearance.

If you have been searching for these answers without much luck, you are in the right place!

Not only will you gain incredible insight in this book, but because I want to make sure to give you as much value as possible, right now for a limited time you can get full **100% FREE access to a VIP bonus EBook** entitled **Anti-Aging Made Easy!**

Just Go Here For Free Instant Access:

www.LuxyLifeNaturals.com

Legal Notice

Disclaimer Notice

Table Of Contents

Introduction

I want to thank you and congratulate you for purchasing the book, *Essential Oils: Quick Start Essential Oils For Beginners And Aromatherapy For Organic Natural Beauty And Health!*

This "Essential Oils" book contains proven steps and strategies on how to use essential oils for beauty and aromatherapy purposes. It is important for any beginner to have a proper understanding of the different methods as well as purposes for these oils in order to be able to use them appropriately. In this book, you will discover:

1. The basics on essential oils
2. The power of aromatherapy
3. The perks of going organic
4. Oil pulling secrets
5. Coconut oil's many benefits
6. Fascinating herbal remedies
7. A new way to lose weight
8. The blood sugar solution
9. An anti aging miracle
10. Interesting cures for pets

As well as other information that you will need to maximize your use and the effects of your favorite essential oil.

Thanks again for purchasing this book, I hope you enjoy it!

Chapter 1: Essential Oils For Beginners

New to using essential oils? Well, there are a few important bits of information that you need to know before you really get started. These would allow you to not just apply the essential oils better but they might even provide you with knowledge that would enable you to take things a step further. After all, there are many things that you can do with these oils.

To help you get started, here are some of the things every beginner should know about essential oils:

- They are not really oils. They do not contain the fatty acids that would normally comprise an oil-based product. However, they are highly concentrated plant constituent which also contains very potent medicinal as well as cosmetic properties. Some people even refer to them as the life force of the plant itself, driving in the point of how potent it can be.

- Most essential oils have very potent antifungal, antibacterial and antiviral properties. This means that besides the usual uses for them, cosmetic and medicinal, you can also add them to your cleaning products. The best bit? It's all natural and wouldn't produce toxic fumes that are bad for your family's health. Some of the best ones for this purpose would be: peppermint, lemon and rosemary.

- Essential oils are actually quite miniscule when looked at molecularly. This means that they are easily absorbed by your skin so their effects can penetrate much quicker and work much faster. For healing and nourishing the skin, they are your best bet. However, it should also be noted that quite unlike other beauty products, essential oils don't accumulate or leave residues in your body even after long time use. Once they've delivered the good stuff, they pass through and out of your system.

- Rosemary essential oil can help you study better. Recent research have shown that taking a whiff of it can actually help you retain more information and at the same time, improve your memory recall thus increasing performances when it comes to test. This is also attributed to the fact that the scent produces calming effects.

- Fragrance oils are not the same thing. Fragrance oils are, more often than not, synthetically made even if it says "natural fragrance". Essential oils, on the other hand, are derived directly from the plant itself and are organic.

- Essential oils cannot be patented because of the fact that they are wholly natural. This means that you'll never be able to find one being used in a pharmaceutical drug. Many mainstream healthcare practitioners won't advocate or recommend its use as an effective alternative to synthetic drugs. Drug companies won't waste time studying them because supposedly, no money can be made from them. Basically, our scientific knowledge of essential oils and their uses is greatly limited. What we do currently know is comprised of information that has been passed down from ancient medicine as well as personal use and experimentation.

- It takes an enormous amount of plants to produce essential oils. This is also why they can be quite expensive, especially if you're going for high quality varieties. To produce a pound of essential oil, 4000 pounds of Bulgarian roses need to be processed. Some do take a little less, such as lavenders which only require 100 pounds of plant material to produce a pound of oil. This kind of processing leaves the oil itself very concentrated, and thus highly potent.

- Most essential oils are not meant to be used undiluted on your skin. Instead, you ought to mix them with carrier oils, butters, waxes as well as any other diluting measures that you prefer. This is because of the fact that they are so concentrated and using them straight can lead to a rather unfortunate skin reaction. Also, do consider if you have any allergies.

Important warnings:

- Want to know if you're sensitive to a certain kind of essential oil? Here's how to test. Combine a drop of our oil with ½ a teaspoon of carrier oil and rub this on the upper portion arm, right on the inside of it where the sensitive skin is. Leave it for a couple of hours. If no itchiness or redness develops, then you're not sensitive to that essential oil.

- Never ingest essential oils, especially eucalyptus and wintergreen. While there are certain ones that can be used in toothpaste, this must be well-diluted to make sure it's safe for accidental consumption. In fact, you must also be aware that there are varieties that can be so toxic, even skin contact must be avoided. Don't fret, however, for these are the rarer ones and you'll never find them easily available in stores.

Chapter 2: Aromatherapy Secrets For Natural Beauty And Health

You've heard of using aromatherapy for relaxation and putting your mind at ease but did you know that it could also be used as a natural beauty treatment? How about as an organic health booster? Well, in this chapter, we'll discuss different essential oils and their effects on our bodies.

- Lemon essential oil. You may think that using oil to counteract oily skin is a little weird but that's exactly what this essential oil does. It helps slow down oil production your skin but without drying it out which is what most synthetic products do. Just rub a few drops onto your problem areas (make sure you dilute it!) and you're good too go.

- Lavender essential oil. Looking for some moisture and nourishment for your skin? Lavender essential oil would be your best bet for this purpose. It is much better than your average lotion because it actually keeps your skin moisturized for hours on end. You don't have to constantly reapply anything. It is also one of the best scar visibility reducer; just rub it onto the area once or twice a day and you'll soon see significant improvement in its appearance.

- Peppermint essential oil. We already know that this has a calming effect on our brains but did you know that it has that same effect on our stomachs. Adding a drop of food-grade peppermint oil to your tea can actually help your digestion significantly, while inhaling its aroma can soothe an upset stomach. For dieters, having some of it handy as an inhaler can help curb the urge to snack.

- Rosemary essential oil. Got dandruff issues? Don't fret! Get a few drops of it and gently massage it onto your scalp; allow this to sit in your hair for at least 30 minutes before rinsing it off with some warm water. You can also mix some of it with your favorite shampoo. A few drops would be enough.

- Chamomile essential oil. The tea version of this is known to induce sleepiness so it isn't surprising to learn that essential oils derived from it can do the same thing. Been suffering from insomnia? Just add a few drops of it to your bath and soak in it for at least half an hour. Not only will your tense muscles relax, you'll start feeling really sleepy after a bit too. Much better than any sleeping pill that you can buy.

- Rose otto essential oil. PMS troubling you? Don't reach for the Tylenol just yet. Give this essential oil a try and massage it onto your shoulders and neck, this would help ease the symptoms associated with monthly pains. It smells fantastic too!

- Cedarwood essential oil. Known to be very healing and soothing to the body, this is great for use on tired muscles as well as for alleviating arthritis. If you exercise a lot then you'll know the pain of muscle soreness after so massaging yourself with this would certainly relieve that. Another purpose it's well suited for would be relieving symptoms of urinary and kidney tract infections. Just add several drops of it to a warm bath and soak for at least half an hour.

- Jasmin essential oil. Feeling a little down and low on energy? Just massage yourself with a few drops of this essential oil and it would help clear your head and bring you to a calmer state of mind. Merely inhaling its scent is known to produce the same kind of effect, perfect for people who have high stress levels and need to wind down at the end of the day. Jasmine is also known to improve the libidos of both men and women so using it as aromatherapy oil is certainly beneficial.

- Geranium essential oil. For cellulites, this would be one of the best oils to use. Take a few drops and massage it onto the area at least twice a day. In about a week or two (depending on the amount of cellulite) you'll start seeing significant improvement.

- Tea tree essential oil. If you've been using natural treatments for your acne (or even store bought ones) then you must have already heard of how potent this essential oil is when it comes to fighting that problem. It is clinically proven to work against acne without causing any damage to the skin. All you need to do is add a few drops of it to your moisturizer or your preferred carrier oil and only apply it to the problem areas.

- Frankincense essential oil. Looking to boost your immune system? Then this is the best essential oil for that purpose. It is both a disinfectant and antiseptic which eliminates the germs in the space where you're in. It can also be applied to wounds to promote healing, and is also able to protect you from tetanus.

- Black pepper essential oil. This aids digestion and at the same time, helps in removing toxins from your body. If you've been feeling gassy, this is also a solution for removing those. It also benefits people who have arthritis and rheumatism by actually eliminating the source of the problem such as uric acid and other toxins that might be triggering the symptoms.

- Cinnamon essential oil. Often employed as a brain tonic, this can also be very beneficial when it comes to treating skin infections, respiratory problems, issues with blood circulation, blood impurity, diabetes as well as menstruation problems. It can even be used to help relieve bad breath!

Chapter 3: Organic Natural Beauty And Health

When you've already grown accustomed to using certain things and products on your body, switching to something even if it is better in many different respects can be quite daunting. This is why it's understandable that some people are still wary about switching to something more organic when it comes to their beauty and health products. However, they are certainly worth giving a try.

For starters, the benefits are quite immense. Once you see things better, you will be more keen on adopting the changes and perhaps, applying it to your lifestyle as well. After all, what could be better than a product that helps you look good from the inside and the outside but without the risk of side effects? To help you understand better, below are the top 5 benefits of going organic.

- Earth friendly. Products that are made synthetically can actually carry a negative impact on the environment. The production of chemical laden beauty and health items also delivers some of these bad chemicals into the water as well as the air we breathe. Keep in mind that all of these things will eventually find their way back to us and will affect us negatively as well. On the other hand, if you opt for something that makes use of natural ingredients all the aforementioned are eliminated or reduced which is great for our environment, allowing it to remain clean and pure.

- Avoid irritants. Typical beauty and health products often contain different chemicals, fillers and artificial colors which can actually cause allergies and irritation in some people. You would be able to avoid all of that and not worry about possible irritants in a product if you choose to go organic. These are the types of products that would work with your skin instead of going against it.

- Protect your nose. Artificial fragrances that are added in synthetic products are used to cover up the scent given off by the other chemicals used in it. So if you think about it, they're using a chemical to cover up another chemical and that can actually lead to something very toxic to smell. In fact, some people get nauseous if they happen to inhale some of it. Organic products, however, don't need any of those things. They are scented naturally using essential oils which are actually good for your health. Aromatherapy anyone?

- You can avoid side effects. One of the most common ingredients used in synthetic health and beauty products would be parabens. They are often used as a means of extending the shelf life of the products. However, they are synthetic and also mimics the hormones naturally produced by the body. This causes worry in some people as it can potentially alter the way your endocrine functions. Some have even said that parabens can also cause cancer. A scary thought, isn't it? But you need not worry about those things if you use organic products. These make use of natural preservatives such as grapefruit seed extract and will not affect your body negatively.

- Better for long term use. Lastly, if you're going to use something for a long period of time then best make sure that it won't leave any bad build up in your body. Synthetic products might be good right now but the more you use it, the more damaging it will eventually be. That's not the case with organic products as these are much gentler and will not cause any damage even after long term use.

Chapter 4: Oil Pulling With Essential Oils

What is oil pulling?

- This is a cheap, safe and uncomplicated procedure that would provide you with a number of different benefits, which range from keeping your mouth healthy to ridding it of harmful bacteria and toxins. It can also be used as a cure and a means of avoiding diseases, helping you live healthier as well as longer.

Some of its benefits include:

- Brighter and whiter teeth
- Healthier gums
- Prevention of bad breath
- A boost in energy
- Fewer migraine attacks
- A clearer mind and better focus
- Alleviation of allergies
- Alleviation of insomnia
- Clearer sinuses
- Better regulated menstrual cycles
- Improved skin health
- Improved lymphatic system
- Lessened PMS symptoms

The best essential oils for pulling:

- Peppermint. This is great if you're looking for an energy boost as well as an improvement in both your mental and physical strength. It is also great for getting rid of bad breath as well as for any headaches you may be experiencing. For digestive issues, this would also be beneficial.

- Orange. Have you been having mood swings lately? Perhaps a constant low mood that you just can't seem to shake? This would be the right essential oil for the job. It can also help in detoxification as well as preventing obesity.

- Grapefruit. On a diet? Well, this essential in particular would actually help you in curbing your cravings and suppressing your appetite. It would prevent you from overeating and aid in weight loss. It is also great if you're experiencing a hangover.

- Lemon. This one is multi-purpose. First off, it's great for relieving cold symptoms effective and quickly. It is also very uplifting, mood and concentration wise. It would also help you in dealing with stress and reducing it. For the body, it is great for detoxification and overall cleansing which should help you get rid of any bad toxin build up.

- Oregano. Traditionally used for treating toothaches, it is one of the best essential oils to use when it comes to oil pulling. It can also provide you with a few other benefits such as: relief of asthma and sore throats. It can also aid in the prevention and cure of parasites as well as viral infections.

- Rosemary. This essential oil is great for boosting the immunity as well as decongesting the liver. If you've been having aches, pains and soreness, it can also help alleviate all of that. It also aids the circulation and cures Candida quite effectively.

Chapter 5: Coconut Oil Handbook

We all know that coconut oil has plenty of great benefits when it comes to both health and beauty. But what exactly are these? What are some of the uses that we could derive from it? Well, to answer all of those questions and more, here's an easy to follow "handbook" that would provide you with all the information you need to get started with using coconut oil.

Health Benefits:

- Heart health. For a while, the misconception that coconut oil is not good for our body was so prevalent that a lot of people missed out on the amazing benefits it has for our heart's health. While it is fat, it is of the good kind and promotes good health. It also contains a significant amount of lauric acid which is great for preventing a number of different heart issues such as high blood pressure and high cholesterol levels. It also effectively reduces artery damage risk.

- Immunity. Coconut oil is an effective immunity booster and helps in strengthening it. Through its antifungal, antiviral, antibacterial, and antimicrobial properties, lauric acid is capable of supporting our immune system when it comes to dealing with various bacteria and viruses.

For Beauty:

- Skin care. This can act as an effective moisturizer regardless of one's skin type. It is, in fact, comparable to mineral oil but without the risks of side effects. It can also be used as a treatment for different skin problems such as dermatitis, psoriasis, eczema as well as skin infections. For skin aging, it is also one of your best defenses as it can effectively delay the appearance of wrinkles as well as sagging.

- Hair care. Looking for something that would provide you with all natural hair treatments? Look no further than your bottle of coconut oil. It would help your hair grow healthier and shinier by nourishing it from the root to the tips. The best bit is that it doesn't leave any build up so your hair won't feel too heavy or greasy.

*Remember to use virgin coconut oil as the processed ones do not contain the same kind of healing properties and are, in fact, not suitable for human consumption.

Chapter 6: Helpful Herbal Remedies For Home Use

Beyond health and beauty, essential oils can be used to treat minor injuries that can occur at home. Below are a few helpful tips on how you can do that.

Treating simple scrapes and cuts:

- For these types of injuries, one would typically resort to using iodine solutions or alcohol. However, antiseptic essential oils can do just as good a job when it comes to this purpose. Diluting oil and spraying it is one of the best application methods. You can also use an herbal salve which contains choice essential oils. These are great and won't burn as much as alcohol does so it's great for younger kids.

- Need a protection for your cut? Some essential oils such as myrrh, benzoin, frankincense contain balsams and resins which actually forms a barrier over your wound. A type of antiseptic gauze or band aid. In the event of an emergency and you have some tea tree or lavender oil lying around, you can apply it directly onto the scrape without diluting.

- The best essential oils for cuts and scrapes? Geranium, lemon, benzoin, frankincense, eucalyptus, lavender, rose, myrrh and tea tree.

Essential oils for treating asthma:

- Most people would warn you against using essential oils to treat asthma, primarily because of the fragrances but it isn't entirely bad. In fact, if used properly and in moderation, it can actually help ease the symptoms. Start with simple body rubs that warms the chest and at the same time, decongests blockages.

- There are also essential oils that have antihistamine properties such as ginger and peppermint. To help reduce bronchial spasms, a whiff of chamomile, geranium, rose and lavender would certainly help.

Essential oils for eye problems:

- The most common eye problems would be eyes strain, inflammation or swelling. Before you grab those pills and eye drops, however, why not turn to the power of essential oils? Chamomile and lavender can easily help in reducing the swelling as well as itchiness. A cold compress that's been soaked in a diluted chamomile oil solution would relax your eyes and effectively ease puffiness.

Chapter 7: Weight Loss Through Essential Oils

Dieting is a challenge in itself, what more with the constant cravings and temptations that are vying for your attention throughout the day. There are synthetic appetite suppressors available but those carry certain side effects that you may not be too keen on risking. So what can you do now?

Go all natural, of course. Through the use of certain essential oils, you can aid your weight loss program and suppress your appetite without worrying about possible side effects.

Here are a few of the best varieties for this purpose:

- Grapefruit. This is one of the most popular essential oils when it comes to weight loss. It helps in curbing appetite so you can avoid overeating. If your diet is putting a mental strain on you, it is also known to help uplift the mind and thoughts. Not only that, it is also capable of reducing cellulite as well as developing, and toning the muscles.

- Lemon. The gentler detoxifier. If you're looking for a way to clean your insides but without having to go through fasting then this is the best route to go. It helps increase your energy levels and can even deal with any intestinal parasites that you might have. Digestive ailments such as hyperacidity can also be managed through regular use.

- Peppermint. Looking to curb your appetite? This would surely help. Just take a few whiffs of it whenever you feel like snacking and it would remove any cravings that you might have. It also helps relax you so if you're stressed and use eating as a release then this would certainly be beneficial.

- Ginger. It isn't a secret that this particular essential oil is great for any digestive issues that you might have. Once you have your digestive system functioning well, you'll be able t burn food more efficiently thus preventing unnecessary fat storage. It can also stimulate your inner strength so if you've been feeling defeated by the lack of results with your diet, this will be of great help.

- Cinnamon. Detoxifying improves digestion, and circulation as well as curbs your cravings. This is certainly a must have for dieters who are looking to go all natural.

Chapter 8: Essential Oil Blood Sugar Solution

Having trouble with controlling your blood sugar? Sure, taking all sorts of medications for it seems like the best thing to do. However, what if there's another solution that's all natural and doesn't carry the same side effects as synthetic medicine?

Well, for that, Ocotea essential oil is the answer. This comes from the Ocotea tree which is part of the cinnamon family; you may notice this from the familiar aroma it gives off.

Here's what you need to know about it:

- It contains a very low amount of cinnamaldehyde. Less than 5% to be exact. Cinnamon contains about 50% of this compound.

- Cinnamaldehyde is the compound that produces skin sensitivity if taken in large doses every day. With Ocotea, however, that risk is greatly reduced to almost nothing.

- It contains some of the highest levels of alpha-humulene and is also a natural anti-inflammatory.

- Alpha-humulene, for those who don't know, is a compound that's known for its ability to reduce the body's response to inflammation and irritation. It is capable of blocking 2 different kinds of anti-inflammatory cytokines.

- It is also known to be able to properly balance the body's blood sugar levels as well as control the symptoms of diabetes. It is also great for treating hypoglycemia as well as stress related conditions.

What are some of the safety concerns?

- There is some concern over non-graded oils being sold so as a consumer; you need to be wary of what you're purchasing. Do make sure that it is a therapeutic grade

Ocotea essential oil. The good quality ones have no known side effects and are regarded as safe for use by the FDA.

- Proper usage. Make sure that you use it properly; diluting it 20:80 (1 part essential oil and 4 parts of vegetable oil). Only apply 2 to 4 drops on the area where it's needed. You can also directly inhale it, diffuse it or take it internally as a dietary supplement.

Chapter 9: Essential Oil For Anti-Aging

All natural skin care doesn't just involve moisturization and protection. There are a number of essential oils that can actually help in delaying skin aging. Here are a few of the most effective ones:

- Rosehip seed oil. This particular blend is known for its potency when it comes to wrinkle prevention. It aids in skin regeneration and at the same time, brightens the skin as well without leaving it greasy. It is high in retinol content as well as antioxidants to clear your skin of any free radicals from the environment which can cause significant damage if left as is.

- Carrot seed oil. This can be used in combination with rose hip seed oil for maximum effects. It can be used for treating various skin issues but also minimizes the appearance of wrinkles while rejuvenating the skin. It stimulates the dermis and helps cell regeneration while detoxifying the surface of the skin as well. Because of its high antioxidant content, it also helps in delaying the signs of skin aging.

- Apricot kernel oil. Often considered a carrier oil, this can actually be used as an effective anti-aging treatment. It contains gamma linoleic acid along with omega 6 fatty acids which helps the skin maintain balance. The oil also has vitamin A and E which is both beneficial to the skin's health and appearance. Antioxidants are also present in it so you can be sure that it's keeping all those free radicals at bay. Lastly, it can keep your skin supple.

- Geranium oil. Often used in many traditional beauty practices, it is very effective when it comes to healing scars and making any spots on your skin fade. Because it improves the circulation in your face, it also makes melanin more uniform and reduces the appearance of fine lines and wrinkles on your skin. It also aids in skin regeneration and keeping your skin's youthful elasticity.

- Pomegranate seed oil. Due to its high antioxidant content, it is capable of clearing your skin of free radicals and preventing free radical damage which is one of the main sources of skin aging. It is also highly moisturizing and helps in enhancing skin elasticity and regeneration while protecting as well as healing damaged skin.

Chapter 10: Natural Remedies For Pets

Just as essential oils are great for humans, it can also benefit our pets both mentally and physically. However, do keep in mind that the oil blends that you enjoy may not produce the same effect when applied to your pets. As a matter of fact, some of these oils can be very dangerous to them, so do take this as a warning.

You can use certain oils in the event of an emergency, such as for first aid or short term use (treatment) of certain conditions that your pet might have. Going all natural with their health and beauty needs can be just as beneficial for you as it is for them.

Here are some of the safest oils to use for your pets:

- Lavender. Considered to be a universal oil, this can be used pure or diluted. Can be used for minor burns, insomnia, allergies, ulcers, anxiety when it comes to car rides as well as car sickness.

- Cardamom. This is a great natural diuretic and helps normalize your pet's appetite. It's also a great antibacterial which can provide relief for coughs, colic, nausea and heartburn.

- Fennel. This assists in detoxifying and breaking down harmful toxins as well as fluid in the tissue. It aids the adrenal cortex and balances out the thyroid, pineal and pituitary glands.

- Helichrysum. A potent antibacterial which can effectively reduce bleeding should your pets injure themselves. It is also capable of aiding the repair of damaged nerves as well as skin regeneration. This can also be used as a treatment for cardiac disease.

- Frankincense. This has been known to help in certain cancer causes. It also boosts the immune system while reducing tumors along with external ulcers. Is also capable of increasing the blood supply to the brain. However, do use it with caution as too much can worsen your pet's hypertension.

- Spearmint. If your pet is now obese, this would help them lose weight by curbing their appetite. It is also great for treatment of colic, nausea and diarrhea. Helps in balancing their metabolism while also stimulating the gallbladder. When used for the short term and properly diluted, it can certainly help with a number of gastrointestinal issues for cats.

Conclusion

Thank you again for purchasing this book on *Essential Oils: Quick Start Essential Oils For Beginners And Aromatherapy For Organic Natural Beauty And Health!*

I am extremely excited to pass this information along to you, and I am so happy that you now have read and can hopefully implement these strategies going forward.

I hope this book was able to help you understand what essential oils are and how these can help you with natural health and beauty issues but without the added risk.

The next step is to get started using this information and to hopefully live a healthy and all natural life!

Please don't be someone who just reads this information and doesn't apply it, the strategies in this book will only benefit you if you use them! If you know of anyone else that could benefit from the information presented here please inform them of this book.

Finally, if you enjoyed this book and feel it has added value to your life in any way, please take the time to share your thoughts and post a review on Amazon. It'd be greatly appreciated!

Thank you and good luck!

Preview Of:

Ultimate Coconut Oil Guide!

Coconut Oil

Coconut Oil Recipes For Organic Skin Care And Natural Beauty, Clean Eating For Weight Loss, Shinning Hair, Better Brain Function And Overall Health!

Introduction

I want to thank you and congratulate you for purchasing the book, *Coconut Oil: Ultimate Coconut Oil Guide! - Coconut Oil Recipes For Organic Skin Care And Natural Beauty, Clean Eating For Weight Loss, Shining Hair, Better Brain Function And Overall Health!*

This book contains proven steps and strategies on how you can take full advantage of the beauty, weight loss and health benefits that coconut oil has to offer. Through this book, you will learn more about:

1. What makes coconut oil healthy?
2. How it can help you get better, more glowing skin.
3. Its effects on your hair and making healthier.
4. Can coconut oil improve your brain function?
5. Weight loss benefits and how it can boost your metabolism.
6. Coconut oil and how it can help treat different illnesses.
7. Recipes for both your diet as well as organic skin care.
8. How to choose the right coconut oil for your needs.

We hope that through this book, you'll be able to recognize the amount of potential that a single bottle of coconut oil contains.

Thanks again for purchasing this book, I hope you enjoy it!

Chapter 1: Coconut Oil For Natural Beauty And Health

These days, more and more people are becoming aware of the effects that chemically manufactured products has on their bodies. As such, many of them have turned to a greener, more organic lifestyle that advocates going all natural when it comes to their food as well as the different products that they use on their bodies.

This isn't surprising, of course, considering the fact that there are a number of illnesses which are associated with constant use of synthetic and often chemical-laden skin and health products. There are certain risks that one must bear when using it; risks which can be avoided altogether if one were to switch over to something that's a bit closer to nature.

The coconut oil is a favorite among health buffs as it is one of those by-products that can be used in a multitude of ways. On one hand, it can be eaten and taken as a supplement which would boost your overall health. On the other, it can be applied topically and used as a beauty product as well as a means of treating certain skin issues.

You get all of these benefits but without worrying about its harmful effects to the body.

Why is it considered one of the best natural remedies out there?

It's all in the composition. About 99% of it is composed of saturated fats (which, in this case isn't as bad as it sounds) as well as traces of polyunsaturated fatty acids and monosaturated fatty acids. Virgin coconut oil retains a higher amount of the good stuff thus it is also valued higher.

It also contains lauric acid and quite a generous amount of it at that. When digested by the body, this would turn into monolaurin and is very beneficial when it comes to dealing with different bacteria and viruses. Diseases such as influenza and herpes are just two of the things that coconut oil can cure in a jiff. A tablespoon of it a day keeps the doctor away, so to speak.

Besides these, it is also one of the most powerful inhibitors of quite a number of different pathogenic organisms ranging from your usual viruses to even protozoa. All of this, of course, is attributed to its high lauric acid content.

For beauty and skincare

Coconut can also be used for cosmetic or skin care purposes. We'll get to the specifics of this in later chapters but to quickly summarize, it is often used for: Hair care, skin care, nails, lips as well as treating different skin issues such as psoriasis. It helps keep the skin youthful and glowing as well as protect it from harmful UV rays.

Thanks for Previewing My Exciting Book Entitled:

"Coconut Oil: Coconut Oil Recipes For Organic Skin Care And Natural Beauty, Clean Eating For Weight Loss, Shinning Hair, Better Brain Function And Overall Health!"

To purchase this book, simply go to the Amazon Kindle store and simply search:

"COCONUT OIL"

Then just scroll down until you see my book. You will know it is mine because you will see my name "Sarah Brooks" underneath the title.

Alternatively, you can visit my author page on Amazon to see this book and other work I have done. Thanks so much, and please don't forget your free bonuses

DON'T LEAVE YET! - CHECK OUT YOUR FREE BONUSES BELOW!

Free Bonus Offer: Get Free Access To The www.LuxyLifeNaturals.com VIP Newsletter!

Once you enter your email address you will immediately get free access to this awesome newsletter!

But wait, right now if you join now for free you will also get free access to the "Secrets of Becoming A Meditation Expert – In 7 Days!" free Ebook!

To claim both your FREE VIP NEWSLETTER MEMBERSHIP and your FREE BONUS Ebook on the SECRETS OF BECOMING A MEDITATION EXPERT IN 7 DAYS!

Just Go To:

www.LuxyLifeNaturals.com